THE 90-DAY
PENIS
ENLARGEMENT
WORKOUT

THE 90-DAY PENIS ENLARGEMENT WORKOUT

How to Enlarge Your Penis in 90 Days
Using Your Hands Only.
No Magic Pills, Formulas, or Devices.
Gain Size. Gain Confidence.

R. Thomas Ferguson

COACHWHIP PUBLICATIONS
GREENVILLE, OHIO

TABLE OF CONTENTS

INTRODUCTION: SHORT AND SWEET

Hello and welcome to the beginning of the rest of your life! If you bought this book, you want to make a change . . . hopefully, a big one. This book will show you how to change your penis with only manual exercises.

While brainstorming how I was going to attack this book, I thought about all the reasons somebody may want to change the size of his penis. After about a week of thinking on this, I had an epiphany. There are a million different reasons a man wants a bigger penis. I could write 500 pages on this topic alone. In fact, every individual reading this probably could write 500 pages detailing his own reasons.

So, I said screw it. If someone wants an easy step-by-step guide on how to increase the size of his penis, than that's what he'll get.

I'm going to eliminate the fluff. By the time you are done reading this book, you will know how to manually enlarge your penis.

Period.

Simple enough?

ACRONYMS AND DEFINITIONS

First things, first. I wrote the chapter about my personal story, intending for it to be my first. Quickly, I realized that it simply could not be written without using some common acronyms and definitions within the world of penis enlargement (PE). Therefore, I'm putting it right at the beginning of the book in hopes that you will take my advice and familiarize yourself with the terms.

Acronyms. Read these! Visualize what you are reading, and understand them. You will need to know this stuff. If anything seems ridiculous to you now, don't worry—you're not alone. When I first started I didn't think I cared about half of this stuff. But you will, so have faith!

Definitions. This is the "glossary" part. It's really just definitions of some words that might show up (e.g., if all you've ever called "it" was a boner, but I'm saying erection . . . now you'll get it!) I suggest you at least skim these terms for words that you might not recognize. At the least, if you are reading through the book and you come across a word you've never heard, refer back to this section and hopefully I've included it. If not, the web is your friend.

ACRONYMS

PE   This will be used in many different ways. It is an abbreviation for *Penis Enlargement.* I will use it as a noun, verb, and even an adjective.

Noun. Welcome to the world of PE!

Verb. When you are PE'ing, it is wise not to smoke a cigar.

Adjective. After you're done your exercises, you'll be thrilled with your veiny, PE'ed dick!

As you can see, it will be interchangeably used. You'll get used to it.

BP   *Bone Pressed* is the penis measurement method used most by doctors and researchers, therefore we will use it in our PE efforts. This is taken by pushing a ruler into your pubic bone above your penis and measuring to the tip. Your friends may have told you that's cheating, growing up. In fact, it is the single most consistent measurement, as we all have different body make-ups. Some of us hold more fat on our pubic bones than others, but portions of that fat can move while humping your female, male, pillow, etc.

BPEL   *Bone Pressed Erect Length* is the length recorded by taking a ruler and measuring from the pubic bone above your penis to the tip of your glans. (If I didn't convince you in the first definition, I should mention it now. BPEL is the only way condom companies do research on length to determine condom sizing.) There will be more on this later.

BPFSL   *Bone Pressed Flaccid Stretched Length* is the same measurement as above, except while flaccid. Push the ruler into your pubic bone above the penis and stretch your penis out as far as possible and measure to the tip. This is one of those measurements I never thought I'd care about, but you'll see why it is important later in this book.

NBPEL   This is the *Non-Bone Pressed Erect Length*. For this measurement, I prefer measuring from the side of the shaft to the tip without pressing into the skin at all. This measurement satisfies the egotist in most men. Think—how much of my dick is actually showing?! If you're a skinny guy, this might not be a big deal to you, but heavier people will have larger fat pads concealing their penis. Hence, we need erect length measurements.

MEG   This is the *Mid-shaft Erect Girth*. There are many different theories on how to take girth measurements. Honestly, it's potato–patotto if you ask me. All I ask is that you be consistent in your measurements. My best gauge was my mid-shaft girth. For me, it was easy to see it was the widest point of my penis (away from the base), therefore it was easy to consistently measure in the same spot and track my progress. (We all look different, so use your own visual indicators for measuring.) *Just make sure they are the same!*

Oh, yeah, you measure this with either a soft, fabric tape measure, or, if you absolutely have no way to obtain that, wrap a string around your penis and mark it off. Then lay the string next to your ruler. I highly suggest a fabric ruler.

BEG   *Base Erect Girth* is the same as above, except measured at your base. For me, I am a lot thicker at my base and it makes it hard to take consistent measurements. So while I'd like to tell you that my girth is almost 6″ (at my base), it's just not consistent enough for me to trust my progress. This is why I stick to MEG measurements throughout. One more time—I don't care what actual measurements you use the most, just use them *every time!*

HEG   I never used the *Head Erect Girth*. I find that I can really swell my head by ballooning (see the glossary), so I did not include this in my progress measurements. I would guess that some guys have mammoth mushroom heads and maybe they are proud of that. If that is you and that's a measurement you want to use because it makes you feel good, go for it. There's no reason you can't track your progress with all of these.

FG   The *Flaccid Girth* is simply the circumference of your soft penis . . . with no erect state at all. I never bothered measuring this as my penis fluctuates far too much. I would not rely on this as a progress-tracking measurement at all. But hey, if you want to measure it for fun, knock yourself out.

FL   This is the *Flaccid Length*. See above, except now we are talking about length. I will say this—as you progress in PE, you will notice what I like to call a consistently larger "flaccid hang." If you've never done PE before, think about the times you've went to use the bathroom. . . . You pull down your pants and you think to yourself, *damn, I look big right now. I wish I looked this way all the time!* If you are consistent with your PE, you will look that big all the time, consistently. In fact, the only time I look smaller is when I'm working out (physically, not with PE). I have my theories. . . .

PI   *Physiological Indicators.* These are "signs" that your penis is giving you as to whether you are working it too hard, not enough, or just right. There is much more about this in a later chapter.

EQ   *Erection Quality* is the quality of your erection. I know, I know . . . no shit. What I mean is that often times you may have a boner, but it is not as hard as it could be. You want to learn to rate your EQ from 1-10. This is going to be a very subjective measurement, so again I advise consistency.
            EQ Values can be given as:

1   A soft, flaccid, limp dick

2-3   A fuller flaccid penis.

4   A decent amount of blood engorging yourself, but not hard enough to have sex or masturbate fluently.

6   Hard enough to have sex or masturbate, but you're not winning any awards for sturdiness.

8   Hard, and something to be proud of if you are having sex. You can push on the skin

and it gives, but it is somewhat sturdy at the base.

9   This is, for the most part, your best erection you will have in any sexual encounter. If you could maintain a 9 all the time, you would be extremely proud and your sexual partner would love you for it.

10 This is the absolute hardest you can get. This is where every vein sticks out, you can hardly press on the skin, and whatever angle your penis sticks out at in an erect state, that's where it's staying without forcing it. 10's are rare. You can force them, but they won't last a while without a combination of all your body's chemistry working together. 10's almost hurt.

The usefulness of these numbers will become clear as you read onward into this book.

DEFINITIONS

Ballooning. Achieving an erection, then kegeling or reverse-kegeling even more blood into the penis to inflate it more than usual.

Boner. Synonym for erection.

Clamping. The act of using a device to hold blood in the penis and restrict outflow. (Not endorsed in this program.)

Classic Grip. Grabbing your penis like you would a golf club, with your palm on the underside of your shaft.

Climax. The point of no return where your body orgasms without your control.

Come. Synonym for orgasm

Condition/Conditioned. The 90 day period in which you toughen up your penis gradually before stressing it with exercises beyond its threshold of acceptance.

Dick. Penis, or a nickname for Richard.

Edema. Fluid build up.

Edging. The act of masturbation (or sex) to keep the penis stimulated just below the point of no return for an extended period of time.

Erection. If you don't know what this is, look it up.

Fat Pad. Refers to the storage of fat on your pubic bone (where your pubic hair is, or would be, if you shave).

Fellatio. Oral sex performed on a guy (blow job).

Flaccid. Penis in a natural, non-erect state.

Flaccid Hang. Positive way of looking at the penis looking large in a flaccid state.

Girth. Thickness of penis, measured in circumference.

Glans. Head of penis.

Hanging. Tying weights to your penis to stretch it. (Not endorsed in this program.)

Hard-on. Erection

Jelq. PE exercise. Using the classic grip, you will grab your lubricated penis as close as you can to the base with your thumb and index finger and grip slightly tight. Slide your grip up to the head of your penis in one slow stroke lasting 3-5 seconds.

Ligaments. Bundle of fibrous tissue that connects the penis to the pubic bone. Stretching these allows more of the penis to hang outside of the body.

Manual Exercise. Exercises performed with hands.

Masturbate. If you don't know what this means, look it up on the web.

Penis. For the purpose of this book, this will include the base, shaft, and glans as one.

Shaft. Anywhere below the glans to the pubic bone.

Stamina Exercise. Exercises that focus on increasing control and delaying orgasm.

Tunica. The outer sheath covering the penis. Enlarging this increases girth.

Turtling. When the penis shrinks to less than a "normal" flaccid state.

MY STORY

As I write this, I am 34 years old. I live with my girlfriend and her two kids. I have three kids of my own. I'm just a normal guy who accidentally stumbled upon a very little known secret . . . you *can* make your penis larger!

Here's the gist of how I came to this conclusion. I had what I thought was an average penis. I measured it a handful of times through my twenties just out of curiosity or sheer boredom. Being the recipient of male insecurities, this is just something a lot of us want to know . . . how do we measure up?

So where did I measure up? Well, I'll tell you that pushing a ruler into my fat pad at my pubic bone, I was just about 6″ erect. OK . . . that sounded average, I thought. Every time I measured (which was most likely years apart), I was still just about 6″. I never made it over the 6″ mark.

Fast forward to about a year after I had met my new girlfriend and love of my life. One day I was having sex with my girlfriend and I thought to myself, *hmm . . . does my penis look large today or what?* I subconsciously paid attention to it over the next few weeks. After making mental notes, my subconscious finally said to my conscious self: *Dude, your penis is definitely bigger than you've ever seen it. What the hell is going on here?!*

So I found some quiet time to myself and pulled out the ruler. To my amazement, I was 6.125″ hard! OK, remember when I said I was juuuuust about 6″?

Yeah, well I was more like 5.75″. So what? I admit it! So in essence, I went from 5.75″ to 6.125″! For all you math geniuses, that's 3/8″ in growth. If you're a woman reading this, than you are saying to yourself, uhhhh . . . so what?! Also, if you are a woman reading this, I say to you, uhhhh, why??? But back to my point, adding 3/8″ to a guy's tool is like adding 100 lb. to his bench press, or taking 10 strokes off his golf game, or earning a $20,000 pay increase.

It is a mammoth achievement!

Except, it was no achievement; this happened by accident, or pure luck, or what? Did the magic penis fairy show up to sprinkle dick dust on me while I slept at night?

I was absolutely baffled, but I was glowing with my newfound knowledge of sporting a shiny new "above-average" penis. We will get into averages later. At this point and at any point, it really shouldn't matter to you. But I'm a realist and know guys have this soul-crushing need to be the biggest and baddest in the land. . . . *sigh.* . . .

So what did I do? I started searching and scouring the internet for how a 30-something year old could possibly have entered Stage Two Puberty (no such thing). What I found out those next few days, and over the next 18 months is what is compiled in this book for you.

Can you go find the info yourself? Sure you can. Did I just make it a hell of a lot easier on you? Sure did!

Back to my story.

I'll cut to the chase. The reason my penis grew was because I was performing a penis exercise known as *edging* without realizing it. What is edging you ask?

Edging in the PE world is this: masturbating for extended periods of time without orgasm. You can finish at the end if you like, but the point of the exercise is to stay at maximum erection for as long as possible. Bullshit, you say, I've jerked off my entire life! Why isn't my penis a foot long?

Again, edging is taking yourself to the brink of climax, then dropping back. Do this over and over and you should see growth. How much growth? Admittedly, not much. Edging is more of a stamina exercise, but I digress.

You see, in my first 18 years of masturbation and sex, everything was quick. Five minutes. It went like this:

START
GET HARD
STIMULATE TO MAXIMUM VELOCITY
COME
DONE

This wasn't very thrilling, and honestly was meant more as maintenance just to get myself through the day. Maybe you can relate.

But now I was with a woman I truly cared for and felt this unbelievable bond with. Our sex was not sex at all—it was practically tantric . . . on a parents' schedule anyway. Every time . . . and I mean *every* time we were together, it lasted from 35-120 minutes. If I had to guess, our median time range was about 50 minutes . . . and it still is.

Now, we all know the couples or the guys who will brag about lasting forever and having crazy sex with their wives or girlfriends for two hours at a time. Shit—maybe they are telling the truth. But here's *my* truth.

We have sex every day, sometimes twice, with the exception of her period. All I can ask is that you believe me. We've been together for three years. We still have sex every day.

In fact, I can put my hand on my heart and swear to God that she has made me come every day I have seen her for the last three years. (The exceptions, I could count on one hand, literally.)

Yeah, she's a keeper.

So how does this pertain to my penis growing? Well, that first year I was with her, we had sex approximately 300 of the possible 365 days. Every time we had sex, I was edging for an average of about 50 minutes.

Remember, I went from 5 minutes or less to 50! Therefore my penis adapted to being swollen to the brink of climax for much longer than it ever had in its life. And it grew!

So now you are saying to yourself, OK, asshole, I don't have a girl that's gonna go for that! Or I'm not gonna sit there and jerk off for 40 minutes a day and hope that I have 3/8″ of an inch added to my penis in a year.

Don't worry—that's *not* what I'm saying you should do. I'm just explaining how I "fell" into the world of penis enlargement.

From my research on why I grew, I found the word *edging*. This in turn led me down a path of non-stop knowledge and an underground sub-cult of people who were performing all sorts of crazy exercises to obtain larger penises.

I was floored. It was working for tons of other men. What I learned, through countless hours of research, trial and error, failures and successes, all led me to where I am now. Here are my two big measurements from Day 1 to approximately 18 months later:

BPEL: 6.125″, Now 8.125″+
MEG: 4.75″, Now 5.375″+

For measurement terminology please refer to the Acronyms section, but as a reminder:

BPEL = Bone Pressed Erect Length (How long your dick is!)

MEG = Mid Erect Girth (How wide your dick is!)

So that's where I stand today. By pure accident, I found the world of penis enlargement. I continue exercising my penis and I continue to grow! The growth may come a lot slower than it used to, but so what?! Since starting PE, I've benefited in the following ways:

Growth. Length, Girth, Flaccid Hang.

Confidence. This is the single most important reason everyone should do PE, whether you want to believe it or not.

Stamina. I can practically last as long as I want, or as long as she wants.

Increased Erection Quality. I have harder boners, and they can last longer.

There you have it. That's a little about how I know what I know, and have benefited from it. Are you ready to learn how you can do it, but in much less time? Say . . . 90 days? Keep reading, and open your mind!

SAFETY FIRST

As with any newly motivated person, the excitement of trying to do too much can definitely be a problem. I can't stress enough the importance of following the program. I have set up the schedule so that you do not overwork yourself. These first three months are meant to condition your penis to receive more and more stress as time goes on. It might seem like the program is moving at a snail's pace at first. But have faith. Less is more, especially in the beginning.

These three months will teach you a lot about your body and how it reacts to the stress of PE. After these initial 90 days you should be well conditioned, you'll have gained a ton of knowledge, and most importantly you will have gained *experience*.

At this point, you will be able to go forth and do more, or continue with the program if you are still experiencing growth. One thing is for certain, you should be moving forward with an already larger, healthier penis.

PHYSIOLOGICAL INDICATORS (PI)
Indicators are basically ways of measuring the overall well being of your penis. If you are new to this it may sound a bit ridiculous, but I assure you it is not. You *can* overwork your penis. This can lead to decreased EQ, a lack of growth, or in a worst-case scenario, injury.

23

Injury???!!!!!!!!!!!!!!

Don't worry! Indicators are fairly easy to notice. You simply need a higher awareness, and you must *pay attention* every day. And remember . . . *less is more!* Do not increase the workload I set forth in the coming chapters.

OK, so what are some indicators? Well indicators can be three things:

> *Positive.* This is a good sign that your PE program is heading in the right direction and you are enlarging and improving the health of your penis.

> *Neutral.* These could be good or bad, or simply mean nothing at all. But you've noticed a change, so I'll try to list those changes or indicators here for your reassurance. It is best to pay attention to these neutral indicators in conjunction with positive or negative indicators to get an overall picture of how you are doing.

> *Negative.* These are bad signs. This means you have overdone it somewhere in your training. If you experience a negative indicator, you need to take a few days' break, or at least back off a bit. The extent of your break will be determined by your own instinct in knowing your body.

Here are some examples:

POSITIVE INDICATORS (PI+)
Increase in normal size. Pretty obvious!

Increased flaccid hang for most or all of the day.

Increased "natural" erections. (Morning or nighttime wood.)

Increased consistent EQ.

Increased sexual desire (horniness).

NEGATIVE INDICATORS (PI-)

Decrease in normal size for more than a day. Again, *obvious!*

Any pains or aches . . . including throbbing.

Numbness, coldness, or tingling.

Discoloration or bruising.

Red spots, broken blood vessels, or blood blisters.

Loss of EQ.

Loss of sexual desire.

Decreased natural erections.

NEUTRAL INDICATORS (PI±)

Temporary increase in size (minutes or a few hours).

Redness.

A few tiny spots.

Achiness in penis. This should not last longer than a day.

Turtling after a workout. *Turtling* is a term for the shrinking of your penis or having a small flaccid hang. Think about jumping in a cold pool. That's turtling.

Fluid build-up or minor swelling. This is called edema.

PI CASE STUDIES

I'm going to share with you three stories of my own. These will serve as examples on how to use these PI's together in determining the state of your PE endeavors and whether to continue or take a break.

Of course, the goal is to keep your PI's positive and not take a break at all in the 90 days. That said, if PE is new to you, you most likely will have some drawbacks. It's part of the learning process. Don't beat yourself up if you have to take a break.

If you are paying attention to your PI's and can submit to some needed breaks, these drawbacks need only be minor breaks in your exercising, and not injuries that require a week off. The choice is yours to pay attention to your body.

In all honesty, I think my ability to "listen" to what my penis told me is the entire reason for my great gains.

OK, onto the case studies:

Case Study #1

When I first started, I stretched my penis for five minutes in different directions. I followed that up with 75 jelqs (see glossary). When I was done, my penis immediately turtled and was red.

That night, I felt a slight twinge in my right side at the base of my penis. I was still able to have sex with my girlfriend. I didn't notice any differences in my EQ and the next morning I was just as ready (erect) as I always am for her.

So let's see what I was experiencing:

Turtling	Neutral
Redness	Neutral
Twinge (Pulled Ligament)	Negative
No Change in Desire or EQ	Neutral

My conclusion was that I was basically new to PE. Everything seemed neutral at this point, except for the "pulling" I was feeling in my base of my penis. I determined that this alone was not enough to take a break, however I just wouldn't pull as hard in my stretching over the next few days.

CASE STUDY #2
Much later in my training career, I tried stretching for an extended period of time. At this point, the maximum stretching I was doing was 7 minutes.

Well one day, I had some free time on my hands and stretched for about 25 minutes.

Afterwards I found I had sore spots at the base of my penis in two different areas. That night when I had sex with my girlfriend, I struggled to maintain a nice hard penis for her. I waxed and waned between an EQ of 6 and 8.

I got the job done for her, but with much stress for myself trying to "keep it up." And that's just not what our sex is about! Hopefully your sexual encounters aren't filled with stress either.

Anyway, the next morning I still felt the pain, almost like a pinching. I had no morning wood at all. When I touched her naked body, I became erect, but that was it. There was no hard-on without the extra stimulation.

I think you are getting the point here without me having to list the negative PI's. I had definitely over-trained, and I was paying for it. I decided to take three days off and told myself not to make that mistake again!

On the third day of no exercise, I gently pulled on my penis and didn't feel any pain, so I decided to give it a go on day four with a normal routine.

I was back to normal after that and my PI's turned back into positive ones shortly thereafter.

Case Study #3
Two months into my beginner's routine, I just completed a workout and decided to measure. *Boom!* I was a bit over *one full inch* in length gain!

My MEG was just slightly less than 1/4″ larger! My penis was getting hard and staying hard in the recent encounters with my woman. (Remember, we have sex every day.) It was starting to look large throughout the day.

Measured Gains
High EQ
Larger Flaccid Hang

All these were positive PI's! It was the green light to proceed with the program. I was doing great! Just think, one extra inch on your penis! This can be you.

In closing, it is up to you to learn your positive and negative PI's. All your neutral ones should be interpreted in context alongside any positives and negatives you are experiencing. Listen to these indicators and proceed accordingly and you will maximize your growth.

As I said before, I think this is the #1 reason I was a quick gainer.

INJURIES

If you religiously follow the plan and pay attention to your PI's, you should not suffer any injuries that would require a week off. What I've found is that the serious injuries happen with people hanging weights from their dicks, or clamping them with actual tools instead of just their hands.

Overusing penis pumps seems to be another injury-inducer, among many others.

The book you are reading specifically does not endorse any of that . . . not because it's a bad idea, but because there is absolutely no need for it in your first 90 days of exercise. These are unnecessary tools in building a larger penis and without experience, can lead to unsafe practices.

So what are some of the injuries you might sustain while exercising with just your hands?

Pulled Ligaments. These are common. I've done this a number of times while being a bit overzealous. This feels like a pinch of pain at the base of your penis where it is attached to your pubic bone with ligaments. This is not the end of the world, and usually it will just take a few days' rest to get yourself back in shape for more PE.

Bruising or Discoloration. If you are not overdoing it, this shouldn't be an issue for you. Remember, Rome was not built in a day and neither will your dick be! Stretch light, squeeze light. If you show up with a bruise the next day, take a few days off. Figure out what you did too hard, and very simply . . . lighten it up! This isn't rocket science. But we as humans *love* to overcomplicate things.

Numbness / Coldness / Tingling. There are probably a few different ways to cause this. The most common would be squeezing too hard, for too long (in a jelq, perhaps).

Again, if this happens to you, take a few days off until everything is back in "working order." See a theme?

Stiff Flaccid. I've never suffered from this. If you notice this happening with you, then it is in your best interest to halt all your PE endeavors until you have a nice soft, limp flaccid again.

Once you attain this, you can start back up under your own advise. However, I'd advise you to start back up slowly. You

are definitely overtraining yourself if this
happens to you.

> *Red Dots.* These are broken blood vessels.
> This is more of a neutral PI, than an in-
> jury. But if you are feeling pain because
> of them, you PE'ed too hard. As with all
> the other injuries, lay off for a few days.
> The red dots don't need to disappear, but
> your pain does. At that point, resume
> your PE efforts.

If you are experiencing some sort of injury that is not
listed here, that's OK. The song remains the same. Stop
your PE for a few days until any injury and associated pain
subsides. Then consider starting back up at a lighter routine (less stretching or fewer jelqs) until you are certain
your penis is back in good health.

It's really a very simple concept. The trouble is that we
always want to take the biggest strides. Taking a break un-
consciously feels like failure . . . like we are wasting time.

If you are going to approach PE intelligently, you have
to be aware that exercising an injured body part does more
damage than good. You have to ride the wave and take
breaks when your body is telling you to do so.

In my first 90 days, I decided to take 3 breaks. In hind-
sight, I missed 5 workouts because of those breaks that I
would have completed if I lived in an ideal world and never
had any issues with my PE training.

Did that affect my gains? Who knows? Who cares? I
still grew. You will too. But you won't grow if you injure
yourself and can't work out at all!

You must learn the most from your mistakes and not
repeat them. Your dick will thank you for it.

WHAT TO DO FIRST

At this point, you are probably growing impatient and wondering what these magic exercises are. We are getting there, I promise. This is all part of the journey and honestly, the exercises are pretty simple. All the information you are receiving now is just as important as the exercises, trust me. Stick with me!

SHOPPING LIST

This is a list of things you will need before you start. They can be from around the house, or you can go purchase them. You'll see why you need these later in this chapter.

A dress sock.

Rice. Just plain rice in a bag.

A hard ruler, without sharp edges. I would not recommend a tape measure.

A flexible fabric ruler is ideal for measuring girth. A string or piece of yarn will suffice, but leaves a lot of room for error.

Some sort of clock. I like to use the stopwatch feature on my cell phone.

Camera.

Lubricant. My favorite is an unscented lotion. Buy an economy size . . . you'll need

it! I would not use baby oil, or any kind
of soap/shampoo product.

STARTING OUT

Set realistic goals. This is where most people have
problems. I'm going to say this once, but you probably
won't listen, anyway: perform PE with the idea of overall
penis health as your goal and let penis enlargement be your
bonus.

Read that again.

Now, go read it again.

You *will* get larger, but how large and how quickly, no-
body knows. We are all different and we all grow at different rates.

Instead of saying, "I want to grow one inch in three
months," try something like this: "I want to see some measured growth every four weeks, or I will change or add to
my workout routine."

Whatever your goals, make them realistic and flexible.
They cannot be rigid goals, because as you pursue PE, you
will learn a ton of new information and you will most likely
see that your original goals need some tweaking.

Take base measurements. These measurements were
all described in the Acronyms section, but let's go through
them again.

First, you want to take measurements under the *same*
circumstances each time to eliminate errors. For example,
don't take your first measurements on Day 1 before your
workout, if on Day 14 you are going to take them after your
workout. Understand? Pick a time to measure, and keep it
consistent.

So what base measurements should you take? Here are the four I suggest:

> BPFSL (*Bone Pressed Flaccid Stretched Length*): You must do this without any erection, so I would suggest you do it first. Basically you grab your penis and pull it straight out away from your body as far as it will go. Your best grip will be right under your glans (penis head). You then take your hard ruler and push it into your pubic bone directly above your penis and measure to the tip. This is your BPFSL. Write it down.
>
> Why is this important?
>
> I mean, who really cares about how far you can stretch your dick, right? I'll tell you why now. As your penis becomes more limber, it in essence is increasing its capacity for holding blood when you are erect.
>
> In most PE'ers, they are able to notice gains in their BPFSL measurement before they turn into erect gains. This held true for myself all throughout my training. If I noticed a change in my BPFSL, but not in my BPEL, it wasn't long before my BPEL caught up in measurement length.
>
> This is a very good indicator of future gains. It is also an extra motivator for you to keep going with PE if you are not seeing erect gains yet.
>
> BPEL (*Bone Pressed Erect Length*): Obviously, enlarging your boner is what you are

shooting for here, so this is probably the most important measurement to you.

Get yourself to full erection and push the ruler into your pubic bone above your penis and measure to the tip. If you are having an "off" day and not achieving an EQ of 9-10, then you should wait until a different day. Remember, we want to be consistent in our measurements, so the circumstances must be the same every time.

You may be asking why you need to press the ruler into your pubic bone. From human to human, weight variations can affect the fat pad above your pubic bone. Even individually, if your weight shifts a few pounds, your fat pad may (or may not) grow or shrink, depending upon the person.

This is the truest way to measure your length gains. This is the way to make sure your penis is actually growing and you are not getting the illusion of your PE efforts either shrinking if you are gaining weight, or working better than you expected if you are losing weight.

Get it? This is the tell-tale measurement that you can count whether you're dieting like crazy, or eating 100 cupcakes per day.

Here is a website to check out, if you are interested in averages. Remember, doctors and researchers use BPEL, as it is a true gauge of penis growth. Warning: This site has cartoon figures of cavemen with boners everywhere. Proceed within the right environment (not while your boss is standing in eyesight). http://www.mraverage.com/results.htm

NBPEL (*Non-Bone Pressed Erect Length*): This is the same measurement as above, except this time you are not to push the ruler in at all.

Warning: This is very easy to cheat! Do not do so.

Unless you are publishing your stats on a local billboard, these measurements are for you only. You are only cheating yourself if you decide to push the ruler into your skin just a "little tiny eeeny weeeny bit."

So, get yourself hard again. Now measure from directly alongside your penis. This will give the truest measure of NBPEL, as more often than not, pubic hair, or just the gradient of skin from your fat pad to the top the base of your penis can skew your numbers.

Why is this important? As far as actual penis growth goes, it's not important at all. As I've discussed, we can fluctuate with our weight so often that even a millimeter of difference can skew your numbers here.

But as men, we all have these huge egos. So we all want to know, well—what do we look like to the other naked person standing in the room, who isn't me?

I guess I should say that this really shouldn't matter, and honestly, it most likely doesn't to your partner. But as males, we will just never get over wanting that big schlong to whip around like a weapon.

So go ahead and measure NBPEL. It might even motivate you to go that extra mile, eat right and exercise, to lose that last millimeter of fat. And let's face it . . . a healthy lifestyle can only help when trying to grow or improve any part of your body (other than your gut).

MEG (*Mid Erect Girth*)

Get yourself up to a 9-10 EQ level. Then take your flexible fabric cloth and wrap it around your penis and record your circumference. I do this at the widest point of my shaft, as it is easy to visually look down and choose where I'm widest . . . even if it's only by a couple of hairs.

This is very simple, but here's the un-simple part: You have to be very consistent in how tightly you wrap the measuring tape. I wrap it so that there is absolutely no space between the tape measure and my skin. However, I will not pull it tight enough to squeeze the skin. This way, I don't measure too low or too high. Be very careful not to skew your numbers here!

Why is this important? A thicker penis will actually increase the volume of your penis a lot more than an increase in length will. This will make her feel "fuller" when you are inside of her.

Is it possible to be too thick? Yes, of course . . . just as it can be too long. But this will vary from woman to woman and what you do with your sex life. You need to be the judge.

If you do not want to use mid-girth in your base measurements, than choose something else girth-related. Whether it be base or glans, or all three measurements averaged out, you should have some sort of girth measurement.

Even if you have a fat penis now and want no extra girth at all, you should take measurements. If you start growing girth-wise, this could be a problem for you and you may want to cut back on girth-building exercises and stick to stretching.

Who in his right mind wouldn't want to get girthier, you ask? Here's a case study to illustrate my point.

Case Study #4

Billie Joe Lover wants a longer penis. He's always had an above average girth of 5.25". BJ *loves* fellatio. His wife *loves* giving it, but she's a very petite girl. As he stands now, she scrapes him with her teeth from time to time, as hard as she tries not to.

About two months after starting PE, BJ is noticing that his wife is really scraping him up. What used to not be a big deal, has turned into an issue. He measures himself and it turns out that he is a quick girth gainer and is already at 5.5" MEG!

To most men, this hardly seems like a problem. But to BJ, he loves his wife and is planning on staying with her forever. She is tiny and just can't open her mouth wide enough to accommodate her husband . . . at least for too long.

So to BJ, this *is* a problem. BJ wants more length, but not at the expense of limiting his sex life with his wife. So he will back off on any girth-attaining exercises and see how he progresses if he just does length-focused exercises.

This is just one example. While a vagina can accommodate almost any width with patience and enough lubrication, a mouth can only open so far.

If you are a fan of anal, large girth is another thing you might want to second-guess before shooting for the stars. Food for thought . . .

Take pictures. My suggestion . . . you should take pictures. This is not necessary. In fact, I didn't take pictures when I started out. I highly regret it now.

As your penis grows, your mind is going to fight you every step of the way. You will second-guess yourself no matter how much larger you look. It will, in plain words, seem surreal.

You will measure with your ruler, and it will show you that you've grown. Let me tell you—the ruler doesn't lie! You will come up with a dozen different reasons why you didn't really grow. But, if you've followed my advice, you most definitely did.

If you still can't believe it, this is where before and after pictures will help. Take them. Hide them wherever you need to. Just do it. You will be glad you did. I wish I could go back in time and see my penis at 2″ shorter, but I can't.

Don't make my mistake. Take them from whatever position you want. These will be for your own use. There is no right or wrong way.

Log your workout. I would highly suggest making a log somewhere. Whether it be on your computer, in your diary, or on a men's health forum. Have something concrete that you can look back on.

It is nice to look back and see what did and didn't work for me. You know what else is great? . . . Having it available when that doubt creeps in that I was talking about earlier.

When I say to myself, you really didn't grow 2″+, did you? I can look back at my log and see my measurements from Day 1.

That is the #1 reason I like it so much.

Oh, another thing. Writing your efforts and progress down serves as accountability. Whether you show it to anyone or not, doesn't matter. Keeping tabs on our daily lives and putting it on paper makes us accountable. This is one of the most useful things any successful person can do in life. This applies to everything, not just the world of PE. So do it!

MAKING A RICE SOCK

A rice sock is needed to warm yourself up before your exercises. What is a rice sock? It's very simple. People have used these as homemade heating pads for aching muscles for a long time.

Here are the steps:

1. Get a dress sock and pour rice into it. This will most likely be messy, so I would suggest over a sink or trash can.
2. Don't fill it up all the way. You want to leave room for the tied-off sock to wrap around your penis.
3. Tie the dress sock.

Easy enough? I'll address what to do with this later when we discuss the actual PE workout. As long as you have it made and ready to go, you're set for now.

THE MEAT AND POTATOES...
SO TO SPEAK

OK, *finally*, you say! This is the chapter where we actually get down to business. I want to warn you—this is not that difficult, and this is not magic!

This is going to be a simple, straightforward system to increase the size of your penis. Everything that led up to this is just as important as doing the actual exercises. I highly advise you to go back and read the beginning of this book if you were overanxious and jumped to this part.

What I'm going to do is break down your schedule into blocks of time. I will lay out sample schedules, but these will only serve as an example.

You *must* tailor them to your own lifestyle, and even more importantly, your PI indicators.

Let me say that again, for the 12th time. You must tailor your workouts to how your penis is feeling and reacting to your workouts. Do not be afraid to be flexible!

Under each example chart, I will provide a blank chart for you to fill in a schedule that ideally fits your needs.

Don't worry. If you can't stick to your schedule, it is not the end of the world and it is not the end of your dick growth. Just keep in mind that if you have to miss a workout, you're still doing more for your penis than you did before you started this journey.

Also, before each chart, I will give an explanation of what you will be doing. You may need to read and re-read these descriptions in regards to hand positioning, penis direction, etc. Make sure you understand them before doing them.

If you do them wrong, technically you are still doing "something," but I put a lot of research and trial and error into how to perform these exercises. My growth is well above average. Give these first three months a try before changing your routine. You'll grow, too.

WARM-UP

Do *not* skip this. Remember the hot-rice sock you made. Before every workout, you are going to warm your penis and ligaments up with this.

Everyone's sock will be different. You are going to have to experiment with warming it up, to get it right. For example, my sock in my microwave for 53 seconds makes it just right. It is hot enough to still be somewhat warm 7 minutes later. Yet, it will not give me third degree burns.

Play with your timing on warming your rice-sock up. Do not burn yourself! After you've figured out what is perfect for you, it's easy. Warm it up in your microwave, and wrap it around the base of your flaccid penis. You want the sock to cover as much of your genitals as possible.

Warm up times can vary, but I suggest a minimum of five minutes. A lot of PE veterans will warm up for 30 minutes or more, reheating their sock as needed. Personally, I think that's overkill, but if you have the time, go for it!

I warm up between 5-10 minutes, usually closer to 7-8. This is an art, not a science. You will tweak this to your own personal needs as you move forward with the program.

Warming up is essential to your whole genital area. Warmed ligaments and the smooth muscle in your penis will be more limber, helping to prevent injury. On top of that, warmed human tissue stretches more, which increases your chances at growth.

Rice sock options: The only other legitimate warm-up I've encountered is a hot shower. That will do the same thing a rice sock will do for you. Feel free to use that instead of a rice sock, especially if you are doing the entire routine in the privacy of your bathroom.

A heating pad is a viable option, but doesn't provide the moist heat of the rice sock or the shower. A hair dryer is a bad idea, as is an infrared light bulb. Any other idea you can come up simply will not be better than the rice-sock or shower. Trust me!

FIVE-DIRECTIONAL STRETCHES

Do these when your penis is flaccid. You are simply grasping your penis below the head (glans) with a somewhat tight grip and pulling with a constant tension away from your body.

There is a "sweet spot" to grab, and you need to find it. You want to feel the pulling in the ligaments that attach to your pubic bone, not in your skin. Your skin will stretch too, but the pull in the ligaments should be your focus.

The timing will change on these as you progress in the program. Your workout charts will tell you how long to do these. I will detail all these stretches by describing your penis position in relationship to your body:

> *Out.* This is pulling the penis directly away from your body. You can do these in any position you choose, but for sake of demonstration let's pretend you are laying on

your back. Grip your penis under the head with a normal grip (thumb furthest away from your body, pinky finger closest). Now pull toward the ceiling and hold it there with slight tension. This should not feel painful. This should feel like a gentle stretch, as all your stretching should feel for these first three months.

Up. This is the same grip, but now you are pulling your penis parallel to your body with the head towards your face. Simple enough?

Down. Now you are pointing it towards your feet. You may want to switch hands, as your grip will get tired. Switch hands as necessary.

Right. For your right stretch, use your left hand in the same manner as above, but pull your penis to your right thigh so that your hand is touching your leg/hip area as you stretch.

Left. Vice versa.

These are the five main directions you will want to start with. This will stretch your ligaments in all different directions, as well as the entire shaft (tunica).

Stretching is a length-focused exercise, but it will serve a bit of growth to your girth as well. As long as we are creating micro-tears in our tissue, the body will repair them larger.

For the record we will call the grip used here the *classic grip*. It is natural to grab things like this, e.g., a baseball bat, golf club, or penis.

CLASSIC GRIP JELQ

This is a girth-focused exercise. This will also increase your length, but for the purpose of these first three months, we are hoping that this should add some thickness to your penis. So what the hell is a jelq?

First, you want to have yourself somewhat erect. Between a 6-7 EQ is ideal for just starting out. (See the Acronyms section if you've forgotten the EQ levels.)

You want to have both hands and your penis lubed up with lotion. Keep the lotion close, you will need to reapply.

Using the classic grip, you will grab your penis as close as you can to the base with your thumb and index finger and grip slightly tight. Slide your grip up to the head of your penis in one slow stroke.

You want each stroke to last 3-5 seconds. This will be difficult to master and will take some practice, but just keep trying. Even if you go too fast at first, that's ok. Just work towards this goal.

The absolutely most important idea of this exercise is to squeeze tight enough to move blood along the entire length of your shaft. This is *not* masturbation, although it will probably feel good. This is focused blood movement. You should have extra blood in your penis from being erect, but not hard enough to limit your squeeze.

One more time, grip your penis as close as you can to your body, than slide your grip slowly along your shaft. Envision the blood moving towards your head and feel it.

Your head should swell. If it doesn't, you can do it better. Keep trying. This might take weeks to figure out. But you will, and no, you are not wasting your time meanwhile. We are striving for perfection. That doesn't mean the pursuit of it will be useless. That is one jelq.

Now grab with your other hand and repeat. Switch your hands back and forth. You want to keep your jelqs even between your hands so that months of this will not cause your penis to start bending in a direction you didn't want it to.

Yes, that *is* possible.

The number of jelqs will be written on your workout charts and are not set in stone. These are guidelines. Tweak it, if you need to.

Pay attention to your PI's!

There will be only a few variations of these exercises, but they won't show up until after the first month. So here is your first month's (four weeks to be exact) sample schedule. You ready to grow?!

SAMPLE SCHEDULE: WEEKS #1-4

SUNDAY	MONDAY	TUESDAY	WEDNESDAY
Make sure you have all the inventory we discussed for your first day. Take measure-ments and pictures.	1.Warm-up 2. 5 Directional Stretches, 60 seconds in each direction. 3. 50 Classic Grip Jelqs (25 each hand)	How are your PI's?	1.Warm-up 2. 5 Directional Stretches, 60 seconds in each direction. 3. 50 Classic Grip Jelqs (25 each hand)
1.Warm-up 2. 5 Directional Stretches, 60 seconds in each direction. 3. 60 Classic Grip Jelqs (30 each hand)	How are your PI's?	1.Warm-up 2. 5 Directional Stretches, 60 seconds in each direction. 3. 60 Classic Grip Jelqs (30 each hand)	How are your PI's?
How are your PI's? Always pay attention!	1.Warm-up 2. 5 Directional Stretches, 60 seconds in each direction. 3. 74 Classic Grip Jelqs (37 each hand)	How are your PI's? Are you getting it yet?	1.Warm-up 2. 5 Directional Stretches, 60 seconds in each direction. 3. 74 Classic Grip Jelqs (37 each hand)
1.Warm-up 2. 5 Directional Stretches, 60 seconds in each direction. 3. 100 Classic Grip Jelqs (50 each hand)	How are your PI's?	1.Warm-up 2. 5 Directional Stretches, 60 seconds in each direction. 3. 100 Classic Grip Jelqs (50 each hand)	Get ready for two days in a row.

THURSDAY	FRIDAY	SATURDAY
How are your PI's?	1.Warm-up 2. 5 Directional Stretches, 60 seconds in each direction. 3. 50 Classic Grip Jelqs (25 each hand)	Have you started a log?
1.Warm-up 2. 5 Directional Stretches, 60 seconds in each direction. 3. 74 Classic Grip Jelqs (37 each hand)	Measure, either after your work-out, or on one of these days off.	Just make sure to be consistent and measure under the same circumstances from here on.
If 74 is too much, back off a little on the jelqs, but don't do more.	1.Warm-up 2. 5 Directional Stretches, 60 seconds in each direction. 3. 74 Classic Grip Jelqs (37 each hand)	Decide if your PI's are positive, and whether you should increase to 100 jelqs. It's OK to wait a few weeks.
1.Warm-up 2. 5 Directional Stretches, 60 seconds in each direction. 3. 100 Classic Grip Jelqs (50 each hand)	1.Warm-up 2. 5 Directional Stretches, 60 seconds in each direction. 3. 100 Classic Grip Jelqs (50 each hand)	How are your PI's? Can you handle two days in a row? If so, the next month will increase. If not, no big deal. Measure.

NOTES

Resist the urge to increase your workout more than is mentioned here. It is not necessary. You cannot rush the growing of your penis. You will risk injury or over-training. Both will be fatal to your goal. Be patient.

Resist the urge to over-measure. Try to adhere to the beginning, middle, and end measurements. If you are not seeing progress, don't be discouraged. Some people take longer than others.

Most likely, though, you are seeing some progress already. Beginner gains can be quite astounding. Hopefully, that's you!

If you can't follow this exact routine, try to follow this idea: three times per week, for the first three weeks with no back-to-back workouts. The fourth week should have four workouts, with one back-to-back, so that you can gauge your soreness and see if you can routinely do double workouts.

If you had negative PI's that are hard to overcome, take a few days off and figure out what you could have done differently. This routine will not be ideal for everyone.

If you can only do 50 jelqs all throughout the first four weeks, so be it. That's 50 more than you've ever done in your life. Don't sweat it.

Next is a blank chart for your first four weeks. Use it as a log, or to pre-schedule your workout if it doesn't fit into the above scheme. But try to follow the plan as laid out.

WEEKS #1-4

SUNDAY	MONDAY	TUESDAY	WEDNESDAY

THURSDAY	FRIDAY	SATURDAY

Before starting Week #6 in this schedule, you need to learn a variation of the jelq. In the first few weeks, you were performing the "classic grip jelq." I call this the classic grip because when you grab your penis, your hand is in a natural position—no bending or wrist-twisting needed.

This next variation of the jelq is actually a much better method (if I were to choose one). Using the two grips together offers a lot of variety in your jelqing workouts.

I would *caution* you not to become partial to one or the other. Each one offers advantages and hits your penis from a different angle. Multiple variations will prompt faster growth.

So here's exercise #4.

OK GRIP JELQ

First go back and re-read the classic grip jelq section. All the same applies to the "state" of your penis, EQ, etc. The only change is the positioning of your hand.

Hold your hand in front of you with your index finger touching your thumb. Your middle finger, ring finger, and pinky will not be gripped. It will look like you are giving someone the "ok" sign. Now keep that hand position and grasp your penis at the base. Read this, and picture it clearly:

Looking down, your thumb and index finger will be the only fingers touching your pubic area (hair). You will not see where your index finger actually touches the tip of your thumb because this will be on the underside of your penis.

The idea is to get this grip pushed into your fat pad as much as possible, therefore being able to jelq as much of your shaft as possible. If you do this correctly, this is the ultimate grip for jelqing. However, I would still employ both grips. It will be easier on your wrists and fingers, and mix up the "attack" on your penis.

You think I'm kidding about the wrists and fingers? I'm not—I had a sprained finger from too many OK grips in a row. It ended up being a nagging injury. So mix them up!

SAMPLE SCHEDULE: WEEKS #5-8

SUNDAY	MONDAY	TUESDAY	WEDNESDAY
	1.Warm-up 2. 5 Directional Stretches, 60 seconds in each direction. 3. 100 Classic Grip Jelqs (50 each hand)	1.Warm-up 2. 5 Directional Stretches, 60 seconds in each direction. 3. 100 Classic Grip Jelqs (50 each hand)	How are your PI's?
	1.Warm-up 2. 5 Directional Stretches, 60 seconds each. 3. 50 Classic Grip Jelqs 4. 50 OK Grip Jelqs	1.Warm-up 2. 5 Directional Stretches, 60 seconds each. 3. 50 Classic Grip Jelqs 4. 50 OK Grip Jelqs	How are your PI's?
	1.Warm-up 2. 5 Directional Stretches, 60 seconds each. 3. 50 Classic Grip Jelqs 4. 50 OK Grip Jelqs	1.Warm-up 2. 5 Directional Stretches, 60 seconds each. 3. 50 Classic Grip Jelqs 4. 50 OK Grip Jelqs	How are your PI's?
	1.Warm-up 2. 5 Directional Stretches, 60 seconds each. 3. 50 Classic Grip Jelqs 4. 50 OK Grip Jelqs	1.Warm-up 2. 5 Directional Stretches, 60 seconds each. 3. 50 Classic Grip Jelqs 4. 50 OK Grip Jelqs	How are your PI's?

THURSDAY	FRIDAY	SATURDAY
1.Warm-up 2. 5 Directional Stretches, 60 seconds in each direction. 3. 100 Classic Grip Jelqs (50 each hand)	1.Warm-up 2. 5 Directional Stretches, 60 seconds in each direction. 3. 100 Classic Grip Jelqs (50 each hand)	
1.Warm-up 2. 5 Directional Stretches, 60 seconds each. 3. 50 Classic Grip Jelqs 4. 50 OK Grip Jelqs	1.Warm-up 2. 5 Directional Stretches, 60 seconds each. 3. 50 Classic Grip Jelqs 4. 50 OK Grip Jelqs	Measure.
1.Warm-up 2. 5 Directional Stretches, 60 seconds each. 3. 50 Classic Grip Jelqs 4. 50 OK Grip Jelqs	1.Warm-up 2. 5 Directional Stretches, 60 seconds each. 3. 50 Classic Grip Jelqs 4. 50 OK Grip Jelqs	
1.Warm-up 2. 5 Directional Stretches, 60 seconds each. 3. 50 Classic Grip Jelqs 4. 50 OK Grip Jelqs	1.Warm-up 2. 5 Directional Stretches, 60 seconds each. 3. 50 Classic Grip Jelqs 4. 50 OK Grip Jelqs	Measure.

WEEKS #5-8

SUNDAY	MONDAY	TUESDAY	WEDNESDAY

THURSDAY	FRIDAY	SATURDAY

In this next workout schedule, I am going to include five weeks instead of four. Week #9 will serve as a "recovery" week. You will be dropping back to 3 days of workouts instead of four. The jelqing portion will also be cut in half.

This will be very hard to do when you're most likely going to want to keep up with the program . . . especially if you have been consistent. But you must take a step backwards to take two steps forward at times. And this is one of those times.

You just spent 8 weeks yanking, gripping, and beating your penis into submission with exercises that are completely new to it! So give it a break. Let it recover and prepare for the final four weeks in your introductory program. I've even included a measurement at the end of the recovery week, so you can reassure yourself that you, in fact, *didn't* lose any gains you may have made already. And if you do lose something little, chalk it up as a mere fluctuation and know that the length/girth will be back—paired with even more gains.

There are two new exercises introduced in this schedule. These are meant to be used as an introduction to two of the exercises I have been using since my initial three month beginning. Both are *great*, and I would consider keeping them in my workout after you are done with this three month program.

Caution: If you are reading this before starting the program, please, please, *please* do not attempt these exercises until they are scheduled. And when it is time to finally incorporate these, follow the small workload of each. Remember—you want your PI's to remain positive! So what are these new exercises?

Here you go:

BUNDLED STRETCH

This stretch is performed like the first of the five directional stretches. Go re-read that exercise for the positioning. Now, for the "bundled part."

You want to twist your penis, than pull it out away from your body. Ideally, you want to be able to twist it a full 360 degrees, than grab securely under the glans and stretch.

This *will* be difficult at first. Holding your penis in a bundled stretch takes practice, and figuring out exactly where to grab for comfort and maximum stretch is trial and error.

If you can't twist a full 360 degrees, that's perfectly fine . . . twist it as far as it will go without pain. You'll get to the full 360 as your penis becomes used to this new stretch and becomes more limber.

Why is this important? With traditional stretches, you are attacking mainly the shaft. Bundling the stretch also attacks the tunica (the girth). You will be creating micro-tears in your penis from all angles with bundles.

When these are on your schedule, you will see that I have split the time in half. Do one stretch with your penis twisted clockwise, and the other half counter-clockwise.

SQUEEZES

These are the first and only exercise in this program that requires a full erection. Or at least an EQ of 8, but 9-10 would be best. Here's the plan:

Do what you have to do to achieve a maximum erection. When in this state, push blood into your penis even further. This is called a reverse kegal. You simply want to squeeze your abs or like you are trying to push out a fart. I know—gross, right? But if you hold yourself in this squeezed position, you should see your glans (penis head) start to inflate a little more than it already is at full erection.

This inflation is called ballooning. While "ballooned," grab as far down at the base of your penis as you can with a classic jelq grip (like a golf club). You are not going to jelq.

Now squeeze and feel the pressure of the blood staying trapped in your veins. If you have a good grip, you will see the veins physically swell. Your penis head should feel harder than ever. Pinch it. If it does, you are doing this correctly. Now hold for the time suggested in the schedule.

Warning: You are going for slight pressure and discomfort. *Slight.* You are not trying to explode your penis! You are not trying to rupture arteries. If you have a few red dots afterwards, it's not the end of the world, but you *did* squeeze too hard. Lighten up for the next workout.

Why is this important? This is an *amazing* girth-focused exercise. The pressure created is, in essence, stretching your penis from the inside out. Jelqs work wonders for girth as well, but variation is the name of the game, so I wanted to make sure you were introduced to a new exercise before your 90 days are up.

After seeing your penis grow, you'll most likely want to keep exercising. Incorporate these squeezes!

SAMPLE SCHEDULE: WEEKS #9-13

SUNDAY	MONDAY	TUESDAY	WEDNESDAY
Easy maintenance week to recover. It may be hard, but give yourself the break.	1.Warm-up 2. 5 Directional Stretches, 60 seconds each. 3. 25 Classic Jelqs 4. 25 OK Jelqs		1.Warm-up 2. 5 Directional Stretches, 60 seconds each. 3. 25 Classic Jelqs 4. 25 OK Jelqs
Two minutes of Bundled Stretches will be added this week.	1.Warm-up 2. 5 Directional Stretches, 60 secs. each direction. 3. Bundled Stretches, 60 secs. each direction. 4. 50 Classic Jelqs 5. 50 OK Jelqs	1.Warm-up 2. 5 Directional Stretches, 60 secs. each direction. 3. Bundled Stretches, 60 secs. each direction. 4. 50 Classic Jelqs 5. 50 OK Jelqs	How are your PI's?
Squeezes will be added this week.	1.Warm-up 2. 5 Directional Stretches, 60 secs. each direction. 3. Bundled Stretches, 60 secs. each direction. 4. 50 Classic Jelqs 5. 50 OK Jelqs	1.Warm-up 2. 5 Directional Stretches, 60 secs. each direction. 3. Bundled Stretches, 60 secs. each direction. 4. 50 Classic Jelqs 5. 50 OK Jelqs	How are your PI's?
	1.Warm-up 2. 5 Directional Stretches, 60 secs. each direction. 3. Bundled Stretches, 60 secs. each direction. 4. 50 Classic Jelqs 5. 50 OK Jelqs 6. 1 minute Squeeze	1.Warm-up 2. 5 Directional Stretches, 60 secs. each direction. 3. Bundled Stretches, 60 secs. each direction. 4. 50 Classic Jelqs 5. 50 OK Jelqs 6. 1 minute Squeeze	How are your PI's?
	1.Warm-up 2. 5 Directional Stretches, as above. 3. Bundled Stretches, as above. 4. 50 Classic Jelqs 5. 50 OK Jelqs 6. 2 mins. Squeeze, 60 secs. per hand.	1.Warm-up 2. 5 Directional Stretches, as above. 3. Bundled Stretches, as above. 4. 50 Classic Jelqs 5. 50 OK Jelqs 6. 2 mins. Squeeze, 60 secs. per hand.	How are your PI's?

THURSDAY	FRIDAY	SATURDAY
	1.Warm-up 2. 5 Directional Stretches, 60 seconds each. 3. 25 Classic Jelqs 4. 25 OK Jelqs	Measure.
1.Warm-up 2. 5 Directional Stretches, 60 secs. each direction. 3. Bundled Stretches, 60 secs. each direction. 4. 50 Classic Jelqs 5. 50 OK Jelqs	1.Warm-up 2. 5 Directional Stretches, 60 secs. each direction. 3. Bundled Stretches, 60 secs. each direction. 4. 50 Classic Jelqs 5. 50 OK Jelqs	How are your PI's?
1.Warm-up 2. 5 Directional Stretches, 60 secs. each direction. 3. Bundled Stretches, 60 secs. each direction. 4. 50 Classic Jelqs 5. 50 OK Jelqs 6. 1 minute Squeeze	1.Warm-up 2. 5 Directional Stretches, 60 secs. each direction. 3. Bundled Stretches, 60 secs. each direction. 4. 50 Classic Jelqs 5. 50 OK Jelqs 6. 1 minute Squeeze	Measure.
1.Warm-up 2. 5 Directional Stretches, 60 secs. each direction. 3. Bundled Stretches, 60 secs. each direction. 4. 50 Classic Jelqs 5. 50 OK Jelqs 6. 2 mins. Squeeze, 60 secs. per hand.	1.Warm-up 2. 5 Directional Stretches, 60 secs. each direction. 3. Bundled Stretches, 60 secs. each direction. 4. 50 Classic Jelqs 5. 50 OK Jelqs 6. 2 mins. Squeeze, 60 secs. per hand.	How are your PI's?
1.Warm-up 2. 5 Directional Stretches, as above. 3. Bundled Stretches, as above. 4. 50 Classic Jelqs 5. 50 OK Jelqs 6. 2 mins. Squeeze, 60 secs. per hand.	1.Warm-up 2. 5 Directional Stretches, as above. 3. Bundled Stretches, as above. 4. 50 Classic Jelqs 5. 50 OK Jelqs 6. 2 mins. Squeeze, 60 secs. per hand.	Measure.

WEEKS #9-13

SUNDAY	MONDAY	TUESDAY	WEDNESDAY

THURSDAY	FRIDAY	SATURDAY

With these 90 days of focused exercises, you should be sporting a bigger, healthier penis. Remember, no two people are alike. You may have grown a little . . . or you may have grown a lot! But this is just the beginning for you. Your penis is now conditioned to handle more workload if you want.

That said, if you have shown growth consistently or recently, I would stick with the same workout routine. There is absolutely no reason to change something that is working. If it ain't broke, don't fix it.

FREQUENTLY ASKED QUESTIONS

CAN I MASTURBATE WHEN I AM DONE?
This is one of the most frequent questions I have seen. This is up to you. It is highly debatable whether or not ejaculation helps or hinders your gains. From what I gather, you want your penis to stay engorged as long as possible after a workout.

With ejaculation, your body's testosterone levels drop and your penis returns to a flaccid state quicker. There is no science determining whether masturbation is good or bad for your gains, though.

SHOULD I ABSTAIN FROM SEX?
This question I think arises for the same reasons that the jerking off question above comes up. It's really about the individual's concerns about ejaculation.

Let me say this in regards to abstaining from sex. Uhhh . . . why? Why would you ever give up a sexual encounter to exercise your penis? That just seems ridiculous and you may need to rethink your priorities.

SHOULD I WATCH PORN TO STAY HARD FOR MY WORKOUTS?
This is a personal choice. I, however, would abstain from porn at all costs. Porn has nothing but negative associations with it. Let me break down just a few reasons porn is

bad for you, and no, I won't go into ethical or moral standards. (To each, his own.)

Porn fabricates the truth, which can give you a dysmorphic idea of the actual average penis size.

Did you know that most penises in porn are only 7"? Eight-inch penises are rare, plain and simple. So why do they look so big on screen? Seven inches *is* big, but do they look even bigger?

The porn industry is a multi-billion dollar industry. They aren't stupid. Camera angles are meticulously edited, and fish eye lenses are used, to make the dicks look huge.

Ever meet a porn star? In most cases, they find the smallest girls possible and even take it a step further by making sure they have small hands.

So this is one reason to stay away from porn. It will give you the wrong idea about average penis sizes and lead you to penis enlargement because of false comparisons. You should be doing PE for yourself; not to keep up with fake-angled enlarged porn industry penises! Seriously, check your head! I had to.

Porn desensitizes you to sexual stimulation.

This is a new phenomenon that you may or may not have heard of, but it has some serious negative effects on people. Since porn has become so easy to acquire free on the internet, it has led to porn addictions.

Basically, if you are jerking off to porn all the time, you could be damaging your whole sexual system. Without getting into the details, here are the two biggest issues with desensitization.

1. Your EQ will suffer greatly when you are with a real girl.
2. You are training your body to orgasm quickly. This is in sharp contrast to the

stamina building you will be doing with
your PE exercises.

TO TELL OR NOT TO TELL?
This is up to you. I didn't tell my girlfriend for a long time,
but she already knew that she helped me put on some size
from the beginning. Did she realize I was getting larger?
Yes. But we didn't talk about it much.

Gauge your own relationships with people before dis-
cussing it. If you know naysayers or skeptics, I would definitely keep it to yourself. Besides, you are already probably skeptical. That's OK; let the ruler show you differently.
You don't need any other pessimism than what you are already naturally dealing with.

HOW LONG WILL IT TAKE ME TO GAIN?
There is no magic formula here. I wish there was. I wish I
could guarantee that you will put on an inch in 90 days. I
would sell a million books that way.

How about looking at it this way: if it takes you a full
year to grow just ¼", your penis is *still* ¼" larger than it
was a year ago. Is that worth it to you?

That's for you to decide, but as you get better at know-
ing your body, you will get better at formulating exercise
plans to achieve what you want. These first 90 days are
your introductory course and should get the ball rolling
for you.

PILLS OR SUPPLEMENTS?
Pills: Nooooooooooooooooooooooooooooo. Do not waste your
money on pills. Pills might have some valuable supple-
ments in them. I won't argue with that, but they are a scam.

Let's back up. Let's say that I'm wrong and 1 out of 100
of the scam pill companies actually works. Are you ready

to take a chance? Especially when all you have to do is some manual exercises as presented here?

If you are still going to take that chance, at least I warned you.

WHAT IF I KEEP FEELING LIKE I AM GOING TO HAVE AN ORGASM WHILE PERFORMING THE EXERCISES?

You need to learn control. Back off until you cool off. You do not want to be ejaculating mid-workout. As your stamina improves, which it will by default from doing these exercises, this will no longer be a problem.

WHAT TO DO NEXT?

Your three months are up and now you should be sporting a larger, healthier penis. Do you pack it up and go back to your normal life? Hell, no!

If you do, you will lose the gains you have made. You need to maintain these gains with some sort of work or you *will* eventually return to what you previously measured . . . maybe a little bit bigger.

If you are like most men, you will want more. If you are still gaining, I would stick with the simple program as long as it is working. There is no need to change anything if you are still gaining. You cannot rush this.

Also keep in mind that you probably had some nice newbie gains. Some of this is most likely due to increased EQ. Most men don't even realize that what they think is a decent boner, is not the potential of their erection.

PE will equate to a much higher EQ *if* you are doing the right things to maintain positive PI's.

That said, don't be dismayed if your gains start to slow a little bit. The actual growth of smooth muscle and tissue will take time. Be thankful for the large, quick gains, but honestly, you can't gain like that forever. Now you're in it for the long haul.

If PE has become part of your lifestyle, instead of a daily chore, than you really won't need much motivation. If you want to research more, there are many different penis enlargement forums out there.

I'll even admit that everything here, you can get for free in these forums. However, these forums are traps. They are overwhelming and have far too much information. They can be very helpful, but I must warn you. A lot of the information is misguided.

Another thing about forums is they are chock full of insecure men. You will waste a lot of time if you get caught up with the drama of every man with a small dick complex. It's human nature to want to associate and relate to others that feel the same. In fact, the camaraderie can be a good thing. But it can also distract you from your original goal of building a bigger better penis.

PE is a very simple thing. Forums will muddy the waters, so be careful. If you are looking for a new exercise because you haven't grown in two months, then by all means, give it a shot. But stay focused on your task at hand.

Used properly, forums can do you good. If you find yourself on them more than once per day, you will become overwhelmed and you'll most likely come back to this book. Why? Because I've given you a straightforward and simple approach to enlarging your penis in 90 days, all while eliminating the fluff, presenting the steps you need in an easy-to-digest format.

Get started!

CPSIA information can be obtained at www.ICGtesting.com
Printed in the USA
LVOW04s1915010515

436906LV00014B/1045/P